First published 2012 by SLACK Incorporated

Published 2024 by CRC Press
2385 NW Executive Center Drive, Suite 320, Boca Raton FL 33431

and by CRC Press
4 Park Square, Milton Park, Abingdon, Oxon, OX14 4RN

CRC Press is an imprint of Taylor & Francis Group, LLC

ISBN: 9781617110443 (pbk)
ISBN: 9781003524700 (ebk)

DOI: 10.1201/9781003524700

Thanks to Medicongress S.r.l. for contributing to the real-ization of this book.

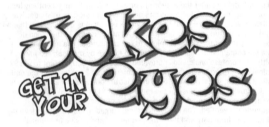

Lucio Buratto, MD
Eye Surgeon
Director of Centro Ambrosiano Oftalmico
Milan, Italy

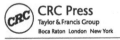

CRC Press
Taylor & Francis Group
Boca Raton London New York

CRC Press is an imprint of the
Taylor & Francis Group, an informa business

DEDICATION

To my friend Johann.

PREFACE

A doctor is a respected professional who qualifies after many years of intense study at university; the profession is associated with an ongoing learning process because of the constant developments and improvements to the techniques and equipment. However, it is a profession that requires seriousness and constant commitment to patient care and well-being. It is an art form as opposed to a profession where honesty, correctness, and loyalty are the keystones of the doctor-patient relationship.

A doctor must respect the severe deontological rules, yet he or she must also factor in some humanity. Consequently, he or she must forge a good relationship with the patient and ensure that the patient is comfortable, particularly when the operations and treatments he or she faces are difficult and extremely delicate.

Sometimes a smile may be the first step toward reducing and dissipating anxiety and tension. And why not? A hearty laugh may even bring some therapeutic benefit. Doctors and patients alike should gladly welcome a joke or a laugh that will bubble up and spill over contagiously to "infect" everyone present.

This book focuses on this unusual topic and I genuinely hope that people reading it will enjoy the humor and take the time to appreciate the lighter side of this serious profession.

—Lucio Buratto, MD

Foreword

Dr. Lucio Buratto is not only a fine surgeon, but he has also written a number of scientific books (*Custom LASIK: Surgical Techniques and Complications* and *Phacoemulsification: Principles and Techniques, Second Edition*) and has branched out into cooking (*The Eye and Nutrition*).

With his latest book, *Jokes Get in Your Eyes*, it is amazing that he was able to accumulate so many jokes related to the eyes. It is refreshing to have a physician who is so well rounded. This book should give at least 30 minutes to an hour of enjoyment. This book can be read by any member of the family; do not worry about its content.

—Robert M. Sinskey, MD
Clinical Professor of Ophthalmology Emeritus
Jules Stein Eye Institute
University of California at Los Angeles

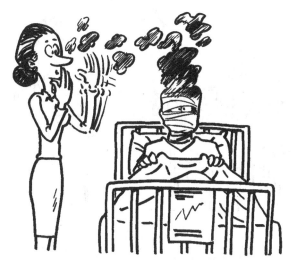

"I'm sorry to disturb you,
but we need some information
for our records. Do you happen to
know whether the laser was the
first or the latest generation?"

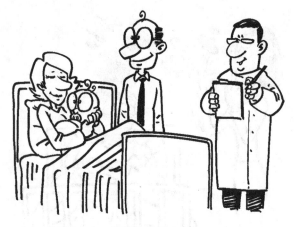

"Oh look!
He has his father's eyes!"

The ultimate satisfaction
for an eye doctor:

To be blinded by love.

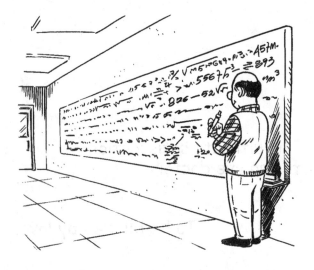

Having the best formula for
astigmatism correction!

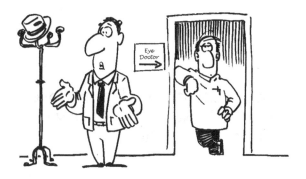

"Well, Doctor, was my
myopia operation a success?"

A man goes into the liquor store and says, "I would like to buy a good bottle of wine."

The cashier asks, "Red or white?"

"You choose. I'm color-blind."

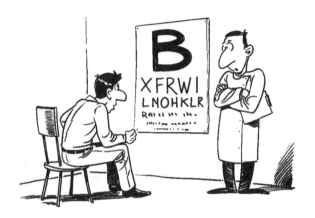

Optometrist: "Read the
first line."

Patient: "M."

Optometrist: "May I ask you a
question? How did you find
my office?"

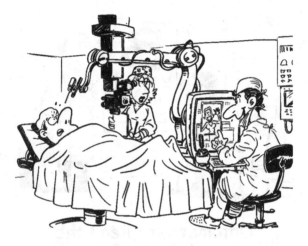

Using computers in surgery.

Doctor: "OK, as we approach the damaged area, you can see... Oh, look! My fiancée is on Facebook!"

Nurse: "Sir, perhaps we should turn off instant messenger?"

He is so short-sighted he cannot even see his contact lenses.

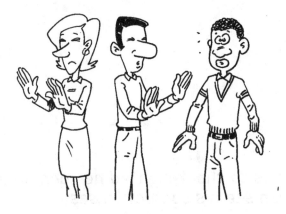

Tom: "I'm upset.
My girlfriend and I find it hard
to see each other."

Ben: "Do you think you will
split up?"

Tom: "No, we just made an
appointment with the eye doctor."

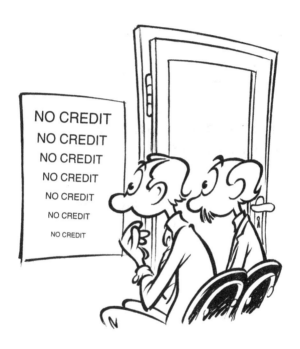

The ultimate frustration for a
one-eyed patient:

To find out that
his right eye is left.

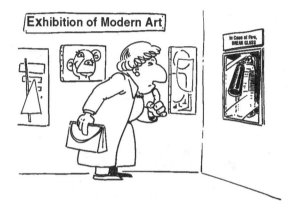

Maybe next time,
skip the museum and go to
the eye doctor...

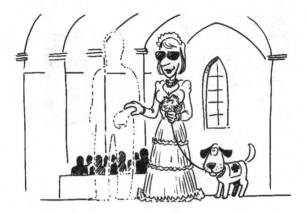

What is the ultimate stroke of luck for the Invisible Man?

To marry a blind woman.

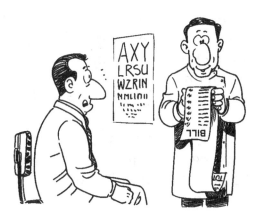

"The good news for you is that
I can correct your myopia.
The good news for me is that
it will be very expensive!"

A pirate walks off his ship. He has a wooden leg, a hook for a hand, and a patch over his right eye. He sits down on a bench and begins throwing peanuts to the seagulls.

Two curious young children shyly sit down next to him and ask the pirate how he came to have a wooden leg.

The pirate replies, "Well, I was standing on the deck of me ship one day, and a wave washed me overboard. Then, a hungry shark attacked me and bit me leg off."

The little boy then asks, "How did you lose your hand?"

"Many years ago, I was fighting the Navy, and one of them boys cut me hand off. Me doc couldn't find a hand, so he gave me this hook."

Next, the little girl asks, "How did you lose your eye?"

"Well, I was standing watch up in the crow's nest, and just as I looked up, a lousy seagull flew over and did his business right in me eye."

The children, now thoroughly confused, ask, "How did that cause you to lose your eye?"

The pirate explains, "Well, it was me first day with the hook."

(Courtesy of George Briscoe)

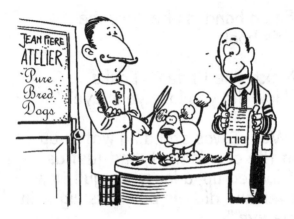

Optometrist: "That's a ridiculous price. I don't even earn that amount as a doctor."

Groomer: "That's exactly what I said to the previous groomer last year when I was still working as an optometrist."

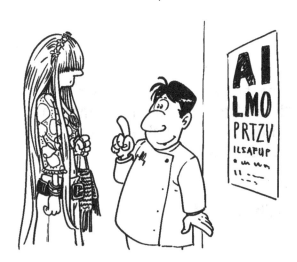

"I think I know the cause of your
eyesight problems...
Do you want the telephone
number of my hairdresser?"

One friend says to the other,
"For the past couple of months,
I haven't been able to run
as fast as I used to."

"Why's that?"

"I blame these tortoiseshell
glasses."

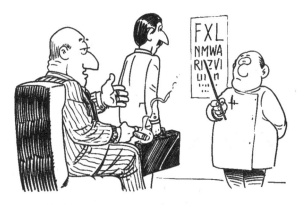

"My attorney will read the
small print!"

Love is blind...

Is there anything the
eye doctor can do?

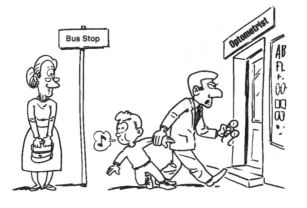

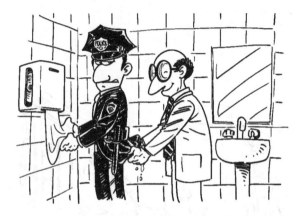

"Maybe it's time you went to the
eye doctor."

He was so cross-eyed that when
he opened one eye, all he could
see was the other.

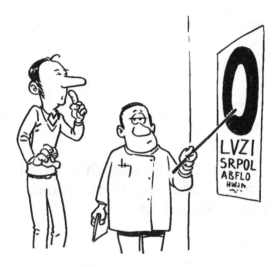

"Give me a clue...
Number or letter?"

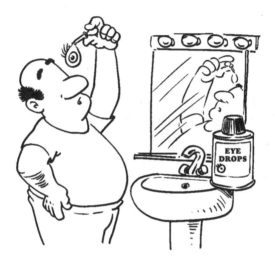

Following cataract surgery,
when the ophthalmologist says,
"See you again soon,"
is he just being pleasant or
is he predicting complications?

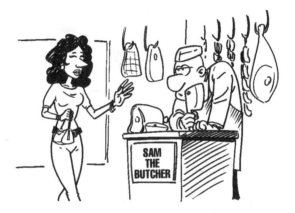

Mrs. Burke: "Please help me! I have serious problems with my sight..."

Sam the Butcher: "I would be happy to help you, ma'am, but this is the butcher's."

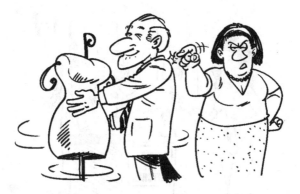

"Put your glasses on, John.
That's not your wife."

For the color-blind:

Are you sure you would be happy
with a vacation in Colorado?

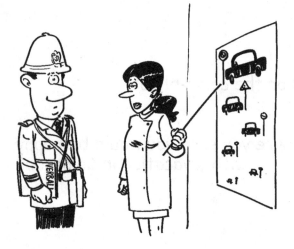

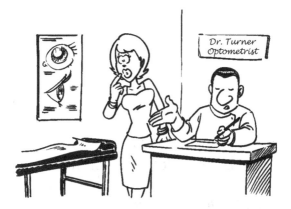

Mrs. Cooper: "Doctor, Doctor,
I've been seeing double for
more than a week now..."

Dr. Turner: "OK, please go and
lie down on the couch."

Mrs. Cooper: "Which one?"

I know I have double vision,
but I don't think I should have to
pay for two examinations!

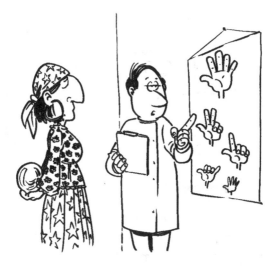

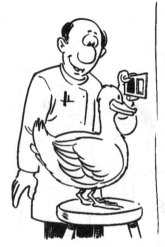
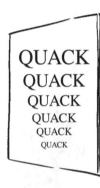

"Well done!
You got the first line right.
Now let's move on to the
second one..."

The ultimate dismay for an
eye doctor:

To be seen in a bad light by
his patients.

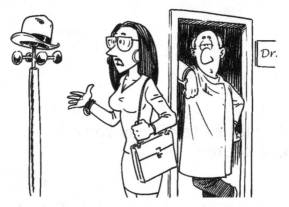

"Doctor, are you sure those glasses you prescribed me are strong enough?"

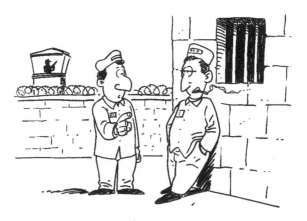

Prisoner 1: "So why
are you here?"

Prisoner 2: "I lost my glasses,
so when I was robbing the bank,
I didn't see the police car
parked outside."

For the color-blind:

Why would you go on vacation to
the Cote d'Azur?

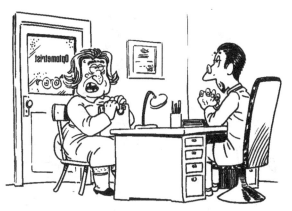

"Doctor, I get really upset when I look in the mirror. I look so old and wrinkly. Can you do anything?"

"There's nothing to worry about, Mrs. Taylor. You don't need glasses—your sight is perfect."

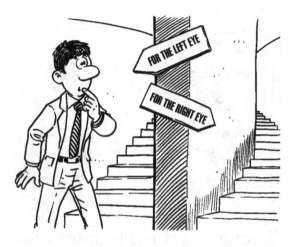

Superspecialization.

A man goes to the eye doctor complaining that he has spots in front of his eyes. The eye doctor prescribes glasses for him.

A month later, the man returns for a check-up.

"Well, are you still seeing spots?" asks the eye doctor.

"Yes, but I have to admit they are much clearer now!"

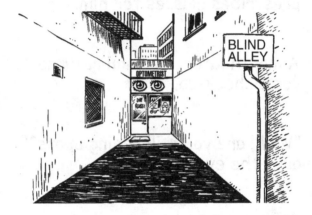

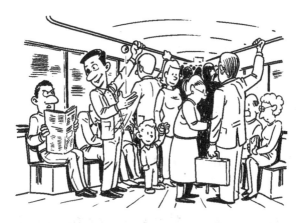

"Excuse me, why are you throwing
your glass eye into the air?"

"I'm just having a look around to
see if there are any free seats."

Love at first sight?

Check with the eye doctor first.

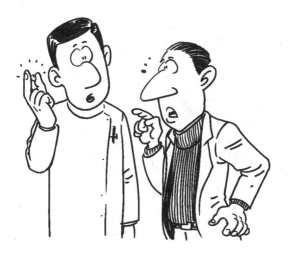

Dr. Johnson: "What do you think of your new contact lenses?"

Mr. Adams: "They look great...
and so tiny...
When can I choose the frames?"

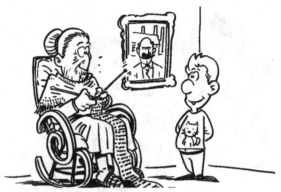

"Grandma, would you close your eyes please?"

"And why do you want me to do that, Johnny?"

"Because Dad says that when you close your eyes, we will be rich."

He was so cross-eyed that when he cried, the tears from his right eye fell onto his left cheek.

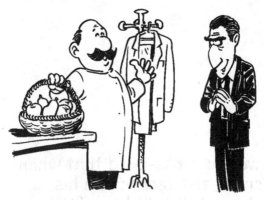

"Doctor, I'm really sorry but
I don't have the money to pay
for my visit."

"Well, you can do what many of
my patients do—they pay me in
kind. The butcher brings me meat,
the tailor makes my clothes, the
baker brings me fresh bread..."

"That's a great idea, Doctor.
By the way, I'm an undertaker."

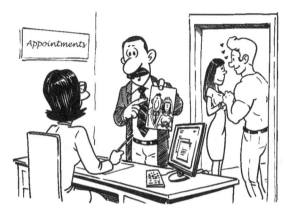

"I would like to make an eye appointment for my daughter."

"Certainly, Mr. Smith. What seems to be the problem?"

"I think she is losing her sight. She went to Spain on her honeymoon with one man and came back with a different one."

"Excuse me, ma'am,
what do I need to do to see
the eye doctor?"

"I would recommend that you
visit another eye doctor first!"

(From the personal collection of Giulio Bozzoni Pantaleoni)

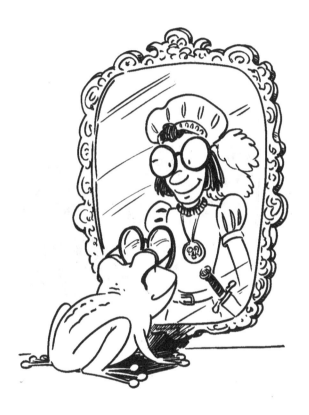

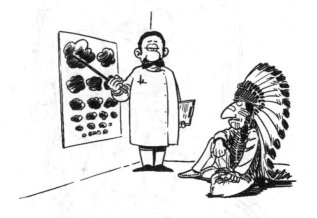

For the color-blind:

Are you sure you can find the
Yellow Brick Road?

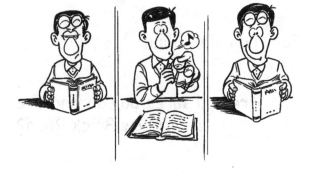

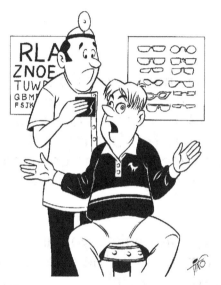

"Doctor, is my sight OK?"

"Well, you are -30 D in your
right eye..."

"I expected that from the
glass eye... Now what about
my left eye?"

After having refereed an important international soccer match, Bob returned home and asked his wife: "Darling, did you see me refereeing the game on TV? How did you think I did?"

"Honey, I've booked you an appointment with the eye doctor tomorrow at 3 pm!"

(From the personal collection of Giulio Bozzoni Pantaleoni)

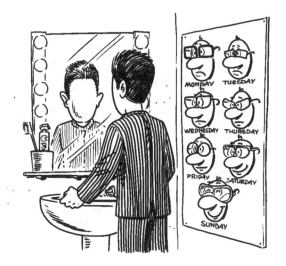

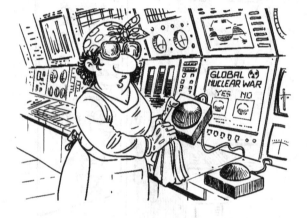

We were not facing each other,
yet our eyes met.

It was then I realized that
we definitely had something in
common:

We were both cross-eyed.

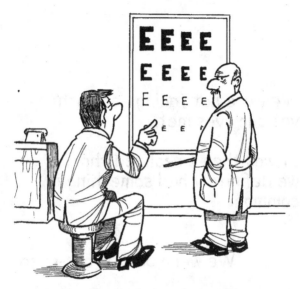

"I'm guessing there's an E in
there somewhere, right?"

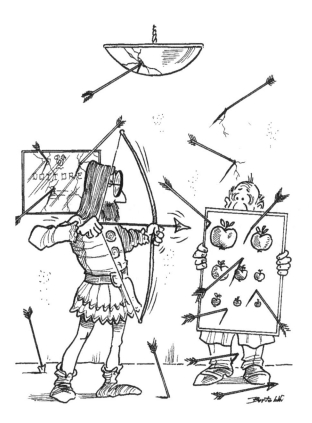

I know I have double vision,
but was it really necessary to
bring in two eye doctors to
tell me that?

(From the personal collection of Giulio Bozzoni Pantaleoni)

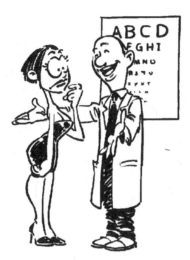

"Mother Nature gave you many
gifts: a clear cornea,
an accommodative crystalline lens,
vitreous with no floaters,
a retina with lots of lovely cones
and rods. So tell me, why did you
refuse all of that and come here
with keratoconus with
a luxated lens and
a detached retina with
hemorrhagic vitreous?"

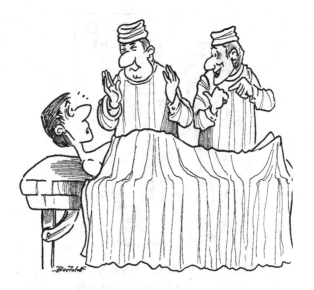

"Now don't you worry.
He is such a good surgeon that he
can operate with his eyes closed."

Following a visit with the eye doctor, the patient leaves the office without paying her bill.

The receptionist runs after her: "I know you can't see very well, but who can I see about paying the bill?"

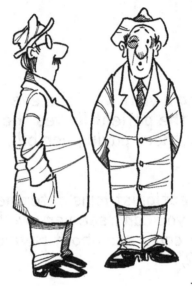

"It's weird, but since I got married I've lost 3D."

"You think that's bad? Since my wife found out I was having an affair, I have lost three houses and got a black eye."

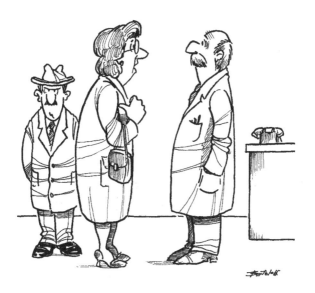

"I know there is nothing wrong
with my sight. I just need
stronger glasses to read
my husband's bank and
credit card statements."

He was so cross-eyed that
he could peep through the
keyhole with both eyes at once.

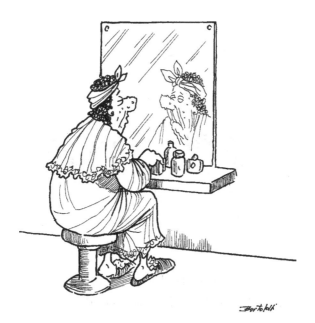

"That's it! I really have to visit
the optometrist. Every time
I look in the mirror,
my face is wrinkled and
my teeth are a mess."

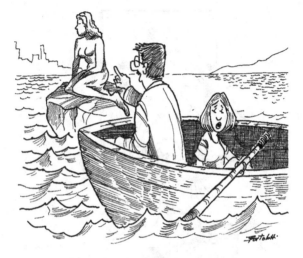

"Judy, if you don't wear your
glasses, you'll damage your sight."

"Hey, Dad, I'm right here
behind you."

The ultimate worry for
an eye doctor:

To be under the
eagle eye of the IRS.

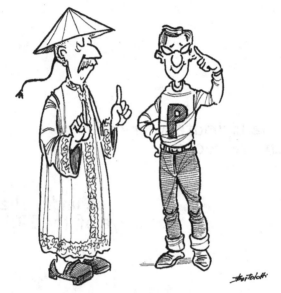

"It happens without you
realizing it. First, you buy a pair
of glasses 'Made in China.'
Next thing you know, you're
wearing a full kimono and
eating with chopsticks..."

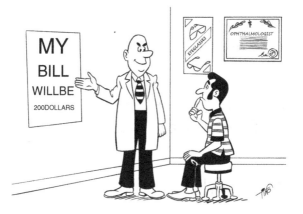

"Doctor, will I see better
with the new glasses you have
prescribed?"

"Of course!"

"And will I be able to
read and write?"

"Certainly!"

"That's fantastic, Doctor.
I was illiterate until now!"

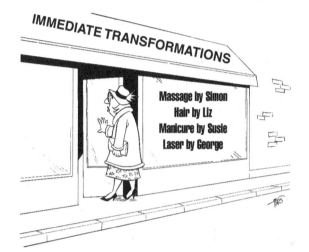

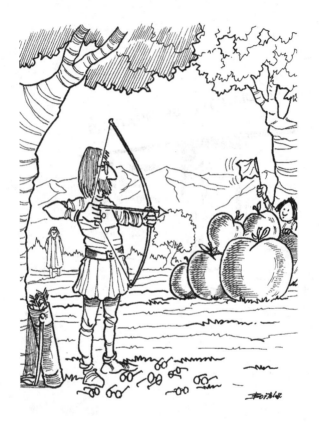

"Doctor, I hope you can help me.
My eye hurts every time I drink
coffee. Is there anything
I can do?"

"Well, for starters, try taking
the spoon out of the cup."

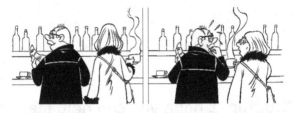

Husband: "Honey, look at that
older couple over there...
guess that will be you and me in
20 more years..."

Wife: "Unfortunately,
that's a mirror
you're looking into."

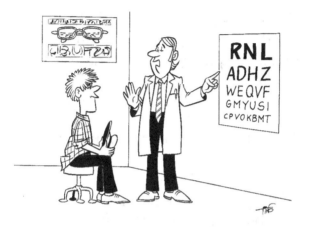

"There's nothing to worry about.
Your sight is fine.
You just need to learn to read."

"Your eyesight is so bad that I will have to prescribe three pairs of glasses," said the eye doctor.

"What? Three pairs? Why?"

"One pair for near vision, one pair for distance vision..."

"And the third pair...?"

"To help you look for the other two!"

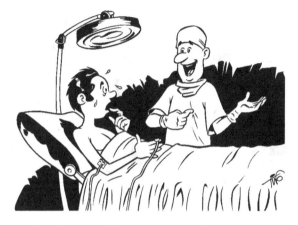

Patient: "I'm worried because
this is my first operation..."

Doctor: "What a coincidence,
I was just saying the same thing!"

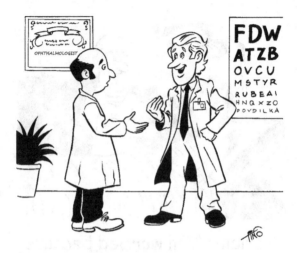

Dr. Max: "How did that operation go on the guy who required emergency surgery for a luxated cataract?"

Dr. Sullivan: "In the end, I couldn't operate...

Dr. Max: "What was the problem?"

Dr. Sullivan: "He only had $100!"

"Doctor, what are the results of my eye exam?"

"Well, you are missing 30 D in your right eye."

"OK, Doctor, that's my glass eye... and the other one?"

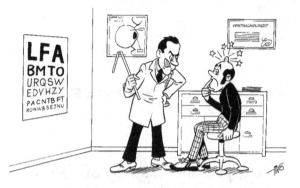

"No, it is not the letter R.
Now try again!"

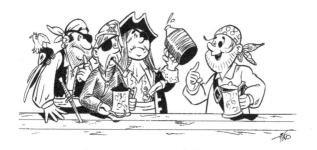

"My eye doctor told me that
my contact patch is the best
he has ever seen."

The eye doctor is a person
who has to keep on revisiting the
alphabet even after graduation.

(Courtesy of Roby Carletta)

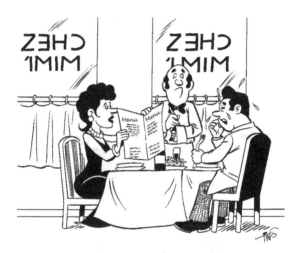

"Jim, you're going to have to admit it: You're presbyopic."

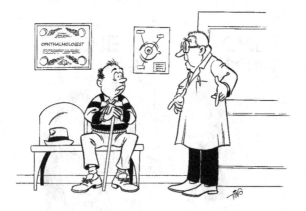

"Hello, ma'am.
You can come in now.
It's your turn."

"Can you read the smallest
letters on the bottom row?"

"Yes, it says,
'End of print run, June 24, 2011.'"

(From the personal collection of Giulio Bozzoni Pantaleoni)

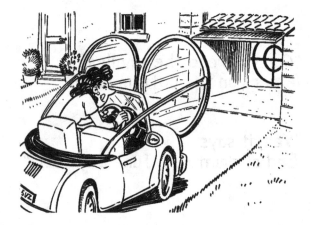

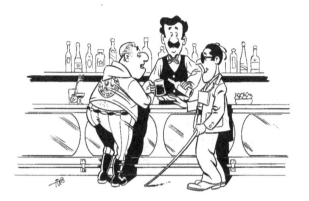

Bud: "A double whiskey, please."

Bartender: "And the same for your friend?"

Bud: "No thanks. He's driving."

A patient trying to select eyeglass frames for himself mentions to the optometrist, "I really like the glasses that Johnny Depp wears..."

The optometrist replies, "Sorry, sir, but I don't think Mr. Depp would be willing to give them up."

(Courtesy of Maurizio Pistis)

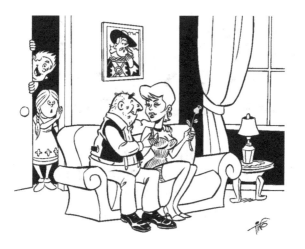

"If that is love at first sight,
we'll need to call the optometrist
for a second opinion."

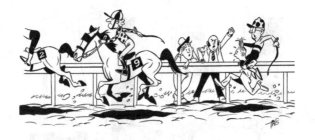

"I don't believe it.
That stupid short-sighted jockey
mistook the stable-hand for
the horse again!"

When I was younger, I had a
friend who became an eye doctor.

Unfortunately,
we lost sight of each other!

(Courtesy of M. Grazia Barca)

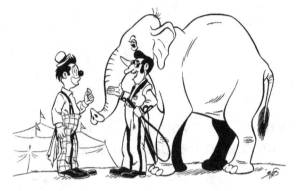

"Weren't you a trainer in the
flea circus last time we met?
How come you are in charge of
the elephants now?"

"My eyesight has gotten worse!"

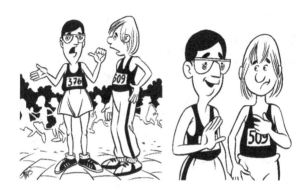

"I have slowed down since
I started wearing glasses.
It must be because they brake."

The man went to see the ophthalmologist at 5 pm. The ophthalmologist was tired and wanted to go home, and he didn't really want to still consult at that time. He asked the man what his problem was, and the man replied, "I can't see far."

The ophthalmologist took him to the window, pointed to the sun, and asked, "What's that?"

The man answered, "That's the sun."

The ophthalmologist replied, "Now how far do you want to see?"

(Courtesy of Johann Kruger)

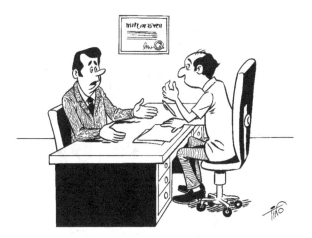

"Doctor, I travel a lot,
I'm frequently overseas for work,
and every time I come home,
I catch my wife in bed with
a different man. Before I have
the chance to say anything
she tells me to go downstairs,
have a cup of coffee, and
come back upstairs in a half hour.
Do you think all that coffee could
affect my eyesight?"

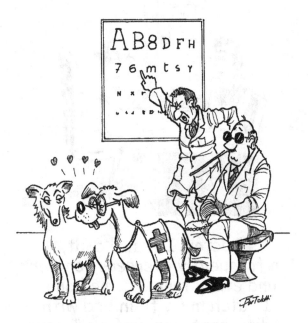

What is the cornea for
a retina specialist?

A shield to the retina for dust.

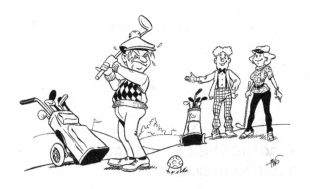

"Oh, dear!
Eddie has forgotten his
glasses again."

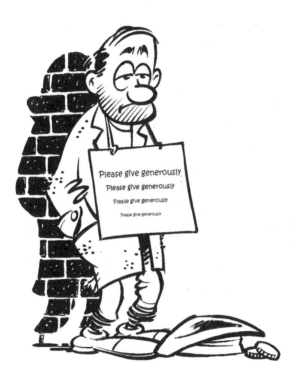

After I have completed the examination and explained the surgery, the patient may reluctantly ask: "What is the worst thing that can happen to me during the operation?"

I look the patient directly in his eyes and think for a moment before replying: "Well, Mr. Jones, I'd say that the worst thing that could happen to you would be for ME to die!"

(Courtesy of Bob Osher)

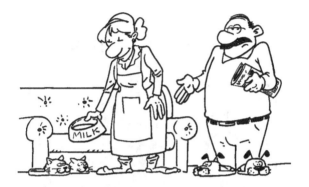

"Darling, those are the slippers
I bought you last week...
Maybe it's time you went to the
eye doctor for a check-up!"

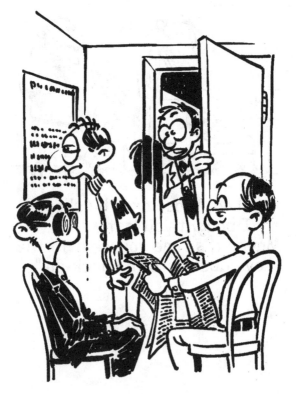

"Excuse me,
by any chance,
is this the eye clinic?"

What is a blind eye following a vitrectomy?

A blind painful eye.

(Courtesy of John Kanellopoulos)

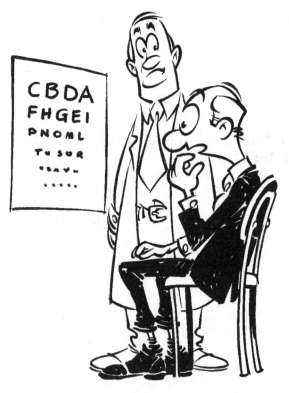

"I'm really sorry.
I'm useless at foreign languages.
Do you have an eye chart
in English?"

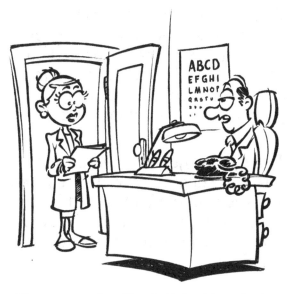

"Doctor, the Invisible Man is in the waiting room."

"Please tell him that I am sorry but I won't be able to see him today."

While my friend was working as a receptionist for an eye surgeon, a very angry woman stormed up to her desk. "Someone stole my wig while I was having surgery yesterday," she complained.

The eye surgeon came out and tried to calm her down. "I assure you that no one on my staff would have done such a thing," he said. "Why do you think it was taken here?"

"After the operation, I noticed the wig I was wearing was cheap-looking and ugly."

"I think," explained the eye surgeon gently, "that means your cataract operation was a success." (Courtesy of George Briscoe)

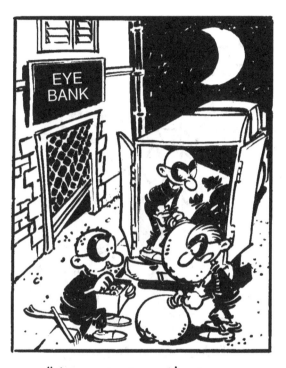

"Are you sure those are
stuffed olives?"

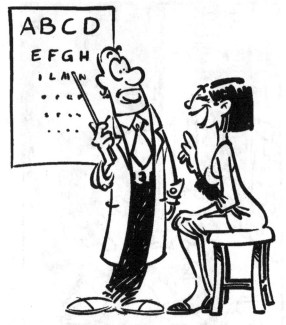

"Now, Mrs. Nichols,
what can you read?"

"Cosmopolitan, People, Vogue,
Us Weekly..."

A man rushed into a busy doctor's office and shouted:
"Doctor! I think I'm shrinking!"

The doctor calmly responded:
"Now, settle down. You will just have to be a little patient."

(Courtesy of Spencer Thornton)

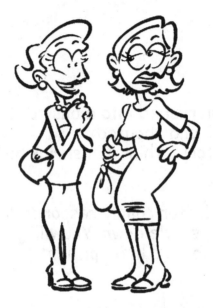

"It was love at first sight
with my ex-husband."

"Well, maybe you should have
given him a second glance..."

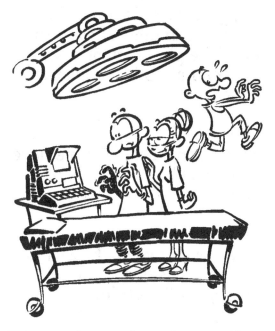

"Now, I know that this is all new
to you, but believe me,
the laser is really
easy to use."

A man goes to his doctor with a sore ankle after falling in the street. The physician opens a drawer and gives him a pair of glasses.

The man complains, "I came here for a sore ankle, not for eye problems."

The doctor answers, "Next time, use these glasses and watch where you put your feet."

(Courtesy of Elie Dahan)

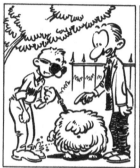 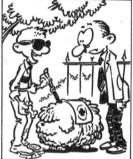

"Excuse me! Your dog has just
made a mess, and
you reward him with a cookie?"

"Certainly. It's the only way
I can find his mouth.
Now watch me kick his butt!"

A 17-year-old boy lost his eye in an accident. He went to the ophthalmologist to get a new eye. The boy asked the price and was upset when he found out it cost $2,000. He said he didn't have that kind of money. The ophthalmologist felt sorry for the good-looking young man, so he said he could make a wooden eye for $500. It would look good but wouldn't last too long. It would give him time to raise $2,000 for the plastic eye. They had a deal, and he had the wooden eye made.

Two weeks later, the boy went to a school dance and was trying to pick out a girl who wouldn't make fun of his new prosthesis, which looked OK but not perfect.

He spotted a girl who had a
hunchback and figured she
would not make fun of him.
He went over to her, tapped her
on her back, and asked,
"Would you like to dance?"
She whirled around and said,
"Wouldn't I, wouldn't I."
He immediately pointed
at her and said,
"Hunchback, hunchback."

(Courtesy of Bob Sinskey)

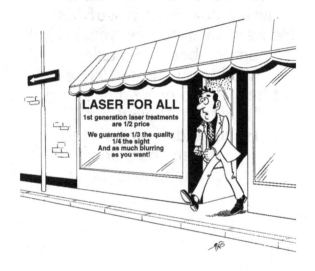

Printed in the United States
by Baker & Taylor Publisher Services